CONTENTS

KU-245-009

UNDERSTANDING BACK PAIN

R.W. PORTER MD FRCS FRCSE
Consultant Orthopaedic Surgeon,
Doncaster Royal Infirmary

*Illustrations by
Keith Reynolds*

Churchill Livingstone

EDINBURGH LONDON MELBOURNE AND NEW YORK 1983

CHURCHILL LIVINGSTONE
Medical Division of Longman Group Limited

Distributed in the United States of America by
Churchill Livingstone Inc., 1560 Broadway, New York,
N.Y. 10036, and by associated companies, branches
and representatives throughout the world.

First published 1983
  Reprinted 1986

ISBN 0 443 02711 0

British Library Cataloguing in Publication Data
Porter, R.W.
  Understanding back pain.—(Churchill
Livingstone patient handbook; 13)
  1. Backache
  I. Title
  616·7'3   RD768

Library of Congress Cataloging in Publication Data
Porter, R.W.
  Understanding back pain.
  (Churchill Livingstone patient handbook; 13)
  1. Backache—Etiology. I. Title II. Series
[DNLM: 1. Backache—Popular works.   WE720 P847u]
RD768.P68 1983   617'.56   82-19766

Produced by Longman Singapore Publishers Pte Ltd.
Printed in Singapore

1. INTRODUCTION

Trying to find your way through the morass of the complex problems of back pain, can be like struggling for a way through a dense jungle. In this book, I would like to try to guide you through. It is not the only way, nor is it necessarily the best way, but I have found a few land-marks which I hope will help.

Stop worrying

Back pain can strike with unexpected suddenness. We are often worried, because it is a new, unpleasant experience and we think it must be very rare. You might be encouraged to know you are not alone, and that only a minority of people go through life without some knowledge of back-

The size of the problem

Out of 100 people in a lifetime
60 will get some back pain
40 will see their doctor
30 will be off work
10 will go to hospital
1 will need an operation
WHY?

ache. Sixty out of every hundred have had back pain; but you may never suffer again because the majority settle down with a little care and common sense; and even with recurrent attacks, they can usually be managed very well without having to seek specialist advice.

Is it serious?

Another common cause of worry is that there might be something very seriously wrong. Put your mind at rest, there is almost certainly no sinister problem at all. Sometimes a growth or an infection can cause back pain, but the type of trouble they cause is not the pattern of pain we shall be describing in this book.

There is also a rare kind of disturbance called 'inflammatory back pain' when the joints of the back become inflamed. It can smoulder on for months or years, but again it is a different complaint to the one we are dealing with in this book, *back pain from mechanical causes.*

What is back pain from mechanical causes?

We may be worried through ignorance. What is really going wrong to cause back pain? We shall be trying in this book to dispel old wives tales, and because back pain of mechanical

Any structure will fail if subject to excessive stress

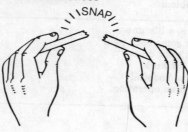

origin is by far the commonest type of back pain, this is the subject we shall be considering in greatest detail.

Any structure will give way at its weakest point if subjected to enough force. The back is no exception. If the load is too great, it will fail at some point, and although some of us have stronger backs than others, every one of us can have back pain from a mechanical failure of the spine, if the force applied to it is sufficiently great.

The body, however, is not a machine, and built into it is a healing process, attempting to repair the damage. Unfortunately when dealing with the spine, the healing may be incomplete, and a permanent weak part of the spine can remain, so that with repeated mechanical strain, sometimes of decreasing degree, the back will let us down again.

This is by far the commonest cause of back pain, resulting from too much force being applied, and some part of the back being damaged.

We shall be trying to explain in this book why sometimes the damage may produce very little pain, how we can go on repeatedly injuring our backs in ignorance, and how other people may produce exactly the same damage to the spine, and have very unpleasant pain indeed.

Will I be crippled?

Another worry is the fear of ending up with crutches, not being able to walk properly, or even needing a wheelchair. What will the end be? Take heart, back pain never killed anyone. You will not be crippled, needing a wheelchair or crutches. If a patient with back pain resorts to crutches, generally his mind is playing tricks on him. Although back pain can trouble us for many years, it does seem to treat us kindly in the later decades of life however severe it has been in the past, often easing up altogether. We hope this book will allay all your fears and keep you in good spirits.

How many causes of back pain are there?

We cannot be sure, because some causes we know and some patients after a most careful assessment remain without a diagnosis. However, the commonest causes of back pain are listed below in the order of their frequency.

1. By far the most common cause is due to a mechanical disturbance of the back. Too much strain has caused some structure to fail. The disc is the main culprit, and we shall be dealing with disc injury in great detail in this book, both in the early stages of damage, and in the later stages when after some years pain can develop from an earlier disc injury. Occasionally the bony part of the spine is fractured, but this is much less common. Pain from mechanical injury to the spine is usually worse on movement when the spine is subjected to strain like lifting; it tends to be eased by rest.

2. A less common cause of back pain is not due to injury at all, but is due to some inflammatory disturbance in the system — the spinal joints become painful because of an internal disease. We shall be discussing this on page 52.

3. Pain may be felt in the back, but have its origin at quite another site. For instance, gynaecological troubles and period pains are often felt in the lower back. Kidney disorders, inflammation of the gallbladder, and some diseases of the arteries can all produce back pain, but they usually are associated with other symptoms which give away their primary source, like heavy periods, bladder problems or indigestion; and the nature of the back pain is generally a constant type of pain unaffected by movements and lifting. The back pain usually represents a minor part of some other more troublesome complaint.

4. Sometimes back pain is caused by a disease in the bones. This, however, is extremely rare and gives a quite differ-

ent pattern of pain to the usual type of back-ache. If the bones themselves are giving pain, it is a constant ache, quite unaffected by movement or lifting or posture. It goes on and on at exactly the same level of pain day and night. This is very rare, can have half a dozen different causes, and can be treated.

We mention these other causes of back pain, mainly to dismiss them, because they represent only a small fraction of the great problem of pain in the back, that is pain largely caused by mechanical failure from undue strain to the spine. In order to understand how these structures fail, we must first learn how the spine is constructed.

2. HOW IS THE SPINE DESIGNED?

There are five basic structures (bones, discs, ligaments, muscles and nerves), and a space called the spinal canal. I hope you will agree that there is a fascinating beauty of design about the spine, with its structure well suited for its complicated function. So often we hear that back pain is the result of poor anatomical design, that man's spine has not adapted to his upright posture. Not a bit of it. It is a miracle of design, and I hope you will be impressed with its structure. Problems arise when we expect too much, and abuse our backs. It is a wonder of engineering which we are only just beginning to investigate, and if respected it should serve us well without problems. Unfortunately, we tend to learn this too late when the damage has been done.

Everything has a breaking point, however good the design, and if you apply too much stress, it will fail. Do not blame the design.

We shall be thinking about the structures that fail, how mechanical strain alters the normal anatomy. Lumbago and fibrositis have been vague terms to describe back-ache, but can we get closer to the mark? What is going wrong? How well do you know your back? A little knowledge of anatomy is essential.

How do the bones in the spine work?

The bones of the spine are called vertebrae, twenty four from top to bottom, but it is the last five, the *lumbar vertebrae*, that are of interest in back-ache.

The twenty-four vertebrae are stacked on top of each other, like a tower of children's bricks. Each one can move a little with the next vertebra, the whole spine being a flexible rod. The largest part of each vertebra is a solid block of bone at the front called the *vertebral body*, each body being separated from its neighbour by a disc. Behind the vertebral body is an arch of bone with three projections, one at the back, the *spinous process*, and two at the side, the *transverse processes* (see p. 8). *Muscles* (see p. 12) and *ligaments* are attached to these processes so that the whole spine is held

From the front

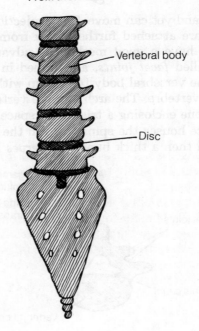

Vertebral body

Disc

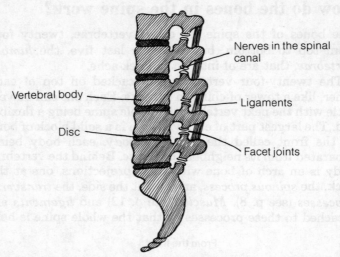

From the side

Nerves in the spinal canal

Vertebral body

Ligaments

Disc

Facet joints

together and yet can move. The projections mean that the muscles are attached further away from the mid-line and therefore have a good mechanical advantage. Two small joints, called *facet joints*, are formed in the arch of bone behind the vertebral body to link up with similar joints at the next vertebra. The arch and the vertebral body form a ring of bone enclosing a triangular space, the *spinal canal*. This space houses the spinal cord in the upper part of the spine and then a thick bundle of *nerves* in the lower part.

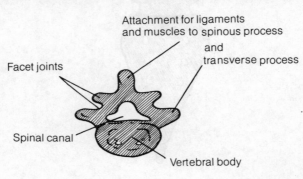

Attachment for ligaments and muscles to spinous process

and transverse process

Facet joints

Spinal canal

Vertebral body

What is the vertebral body?

The vertebrae conveniently get bigger towards the bottom of the spine and are therefore well able to take the increasing forces, — the last lumbar vertebra being particularly strong, supporting the rest of the spine above it.

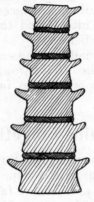

Largest vertebral bodies at bottom of spine

It is the vertebral body that takes most of the load, but there is a limit to what it can stand.

If you fall from a height or are ejected from a pilot's seat in an aeroplane, the vertical compression force on the vertebral body can cause a fracture of the vertebral body. It becomes squashed and the spine very slightly bent.

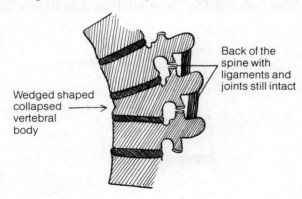

Wedged shaped collapsed vertebral body

Back of the spine with ligaments and joints still intact

This same fracture can occur in older ladies if their bones become very soft, when even the normal stresses on the spine can cause a vertebral body to collapse. This is far less serious than it sounds, however. After a few weeks of discomfort, the pain settles, and usually no disability remains at all. This is because the structures at the back of the spine have not been disturbed. The facet joints, the ligaments and muscles are all intact, and the spine quickly becomes as strong as it was before.

The vertebral body is normally strong enough to take all the stresses and strains applied to it throughout a lifetime, unless you are unfortunate enough to fall like Humpty Dumpty, from a high wall.

How are the bones joined together?

Each vertebra is linked to the next by a three joint system. One joint is the large disc of gristle joining the vertebral bodies together at the front, and the two facet joints at the back complete the system. These two facet joints allow some spinal movement, but are so shaped that they also act as restrainers of movement. They permit us to bend forwards and touch our toes, and to lean backwards. They allow some sideways movement, but are so designed that very little twisting movement is possible in the lumbar spine. The twisting that is possible occurs higher up the back.

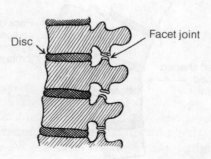

Disc   Facet joint

If the facet joints did not restrain this twisting movement, the disc could be irreparably damaged. In fact, a few of us are born with misshapen facet joints which may be a factor in placing extra stress on the disc when we twist — one reason why some of us are prone to disc injury.

If the joint is damaged, then gradually over the years the surfaces of the facet joints can wear down, become rough and irregular, and give rise to back pain.

Sometimes even a sharp twist can fracture the edge of a facet joint, and produce sudden pain. The diagnosis is difficult because this fracture is not easily seen on X-ray.

What are ligaments?

Most people think of ligaments as ropes, holding structures together as a guy rope will hold up the mast of a ship. Indeed, in some parts of the body this is true. In the spine, however, the ligaments are active, not passive structures, because muscles are attached to them, altering their tension.

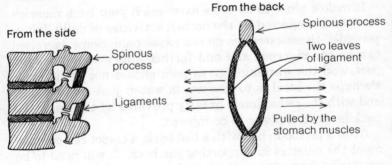

The spinal ligament for example is a strong ligament at the back of the spine, between the spinous processes. It is split into two leaves, which separate from each other when stretched by the pull of the stomach muscles. If we are lifting a weight in the stooped position, we unconsciously

11

contract the stomach muscles. These pull on the leaves of the spinal ligament, and with the minimum of force prevent too much separation of the spinous processes, which in turn could have damaged a disc.

It makes sense to keep the stomach muscles strong if we want a good back for lifting.

How do muscles work in supporting the spine?

We must think about the muscles that support the spine, in addition to the bones themselves, because the spine is designed not only for support but also for movement. Normal activities such as walking and running, lifting and bending, keep the spinal muscles in tone without the need for any special exercises. We do know, however, that if we do not use a muscle it will quickly lose half its strength. A couple of weeks in bed can very quickly produce a weak back. Not a few patients first injure their back after getting up from some other illness.

It makes sense to do some exercises if your back muscles have been neglected by the normal activities of daily living, provided those exercises do not cause pain. Some exercises can be too vigorous and add further injury to a damaged part, and the warning sign of pain should not be ignored. Perhaps the ideal is to exercise in water; just swim about, and with the reduction in gravity provided by the water the back is most unlikely to be injured.

After a period in bed with a bad back, a corset can complement the muscles in supporting the back. It will need to be gradually discarded as the muscles regain their strength.

An important space within the bone

The spinal canal is a space within the back of the vertebra. It forms a segmental tube behind the vertebral bodies and the discs. It is a very important space because, within, it contains the spinal cord in the upper part of the spine, and a bundle of spinal nerves in the lower lumbar part of the spine.

The spinal nerves float about in spinal fluid all of which is enclosed in a membrane, the dura. They normally have plenty of room to move in the spinal fluid. A pair of nerves leave the spine at each vertebra, one on either side.

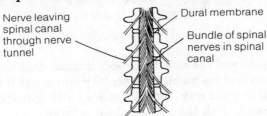

Nerve leaving spinal canal through nerve tunnel

Dural membrane

Bundle of spinal nerves in spinal canal

Millions of messages pass along these nerves each day, giving the brain information about the limbs, and transmitting impulses for movement. Therefore a highly important concentration of nervous tissue is present at the lower lumbar spine. It can be considered the 'spaghetti junction' of the nervous system, the highway for all the nerves of the lower part of the body; the size of this space is therefore significant.

We all have individual differences, both in our size and our shape. Not only do our faces and fingerprints differ, but no two of us have an absolutely identical anatomy.

The spinal canal is no exception. It has a different cross-sectional area and shape for each one of us. Some have a wide canal shaped like a bell, others have a canal like a pirate's hat.

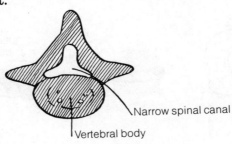

Narrow spinal canal

Vertebral body

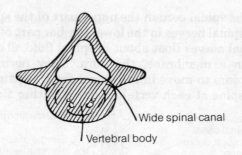

Wide spinal canal

Vertebral body

The shape and the size of the spinal canal does not matter at all, provided we maintain a healthy spine, but if the back is injured in some way, the nerves in a small spinal canal are much more at risk than if the canal is large.

What is a disc?

The centre of the disc is composed of soft jelly-like material called the *nucleus*. It gradually merges with the tough outer part, the *annulus*. This structure allows a certain amount of movement to take place between the vertebrae, with the soft central nucleus moving slightly from side to side and front to back with spinal movement.

The annulus has an interesting laminated construction, with layer upon layer of fibres, like the layers of an onion. The fibres of one layer lie in a slanting direction, whilst those of the next layer will be in the opposite oblique direction. We have designed the radial motor car tyre in the same way. It enables enormous compression forces to be

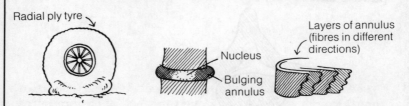

Radial ply tyre

Nucleus

Bulging annulus

Layers of annulus (fibres in different directions)

contained. The laminated structure will bulge but not give way. Besides permitting spinal movement, the discs act as shock-absorbers.

How does a disc work and what is it made of?

Compression forces are so efficiently absorbed by the disc, that the bone of the vertebral body will give way and fracture before the disc is damaged. If we fall from a height and land on our feet, we are more likely to fracture the spine than injure a disc, and fortunately this is a type of fracture that heals without leaving disability. Weight lifters can safely lift 200 kg and provided the spine is straight, the annulus will take the strain, and the disc will merely bulge.

The disc is composed mainly of water and a protein. The nutrition of the disc depends on oxygen and nutriments entering the disc as water exchanges from the surrounding tissues. Waste products are removed from the disc by the same movement of water. We know about two forces which control this flow of fluid.

1. There is a pressure which drives fluid out of the disc, *hydrostatic pressure*. This is caused by the weight of the body and muscle pressure squeezing fluid out of the disc.
2. There is a pressure which sucks fluid into the disc, *osmotic pressure*. It is the protein with an affinity for water that sucks the fluid towards it.

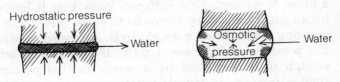

The amount of fluid in the disc depends upon a balance of these two pressures. At any one time, one of the pressures may be stronger. For instance, after lying in bed all night, the discs are slightly more swollen, and it is common knowledge that we are a little taller in the morning. It is because the reduced hydrostatic pressure, reducing the pressure on the discs when we lie down, allows the unopposed osmotic pressure to suck in water into the discs at night. Perhaps that is why we waken with a stiff back in the morning. Similarly, astronauts return from a weightless journey in space with swollen discs, and find themselves a centimeter or two taller.

It is important to appreciate the pressures inside a disc, especially if that disc has already been partially damaged. The pressure can build up to a sufficient level for the central nucleus to be squeezed out of a weakened annulus.

There are two other factors that affect the pressure in the disc, firstly the posture we adopt, and secondly the load we carry. The least pressure of all in the disc is recorded when we lie down on the floor, lying on our back with the hips and knees bent at a right angle, the calfs of our legs resting on two or three pillows. Try this position if you are suddenly seized with a spasm of severe back pain. The pressure

If pain is severe

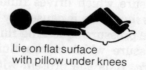

Lie on flat surface
with pillow under knees

increases as we stand up, and is greater if we stoop forwards a little. Most back pain sufferers know that it hurts their backs when they stoop forwards to clean their teeth in the morning. Start lifting a weight in this stooped position and the pressure really rises. Lastly, if you are unfortunate enough to be surprised by a sneeze in this posture, the sudden increase in muscle pressure so increases the disc pressure that if there is a weakness of the outer rim of the annulus, the central nucleus can hardly help but be squeezed out into the spinal canal.

If all this discussion about pressures seems complicated, it is nevertheless important, because it makes sense of our common observations about back pain.

17

3. HOW DO WE INJURE A DISC?

Inherent weakness

Some people are more prone to damage a disc than others. They may have a very quiet job, put little stress on the spine, and yet damage a disc. Such people often find that disc injury and back pain runs in the family. They have a weakness or a small fissure in the annulus, which may amount only to a small bulge when the nucleus is under pressure.

A large mechanical force, however, can convert the weakened annulus into a tear, allowing the nucleus to rupture through the tear.

If we are born with a weakened annulus, it will not take much strain to damage the disc. If we are fortunate enough to have a strong annulus, we may find we can abuse our backs for a lifetime without damaging the disc at all. And there is a gradation of disc strength between these two extremes.

Can twisting damage a disc?

Even if the disc has an inherent weakness, with part of the disc tending to bulge under pressure, it is not usually a compression force that finally tears the annulus. The arrangement of the laminated annular fibres keeps the disc intact under compression, but if a twisting force is added to this it produces a tear. During a twisting motion, one layer of the annular fibres will relax, but the next layer will be stretched. Six degrees of rotation will irreversibly stretch the fibres, and sixteen degrees will tear them.

The facet joints at the back of the vertebrae prevent too much rotation taking place, but if we bend forwards, these joints become less securely engaged allowing more rotation. Thus the damage is likely to occur when we are bent forwards, lifting something to compress the disc, and then if we add to this a twist, the disc is torn. Lifting a baby out of a cot, or a sack of potatoes from the boot of a car will do the damage.

Once the annulus is torn, there is nothing to stop the nucleus pushing its way through the rent. Suddenly or slowly over many weeks, the nucleus is squeezed out through the hole.

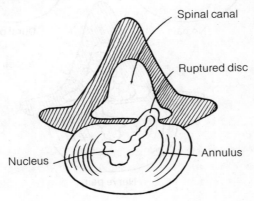

Spinal canal

Ruptured disc

Annulus

Nucleus

What is the cause of disc symptoms?

The disc's weakest place is at the back, so when it bulges or ruptures it does so towards the spinal canal. It is usually to one or other side, because in the mid-line is a tough ligament. It is possible for the damaged disc to cause no trouble at all. The nerves within their dural sheath just move out of harm's way. It is true that years later the effects of a previously silent damaged disc declare themselves, but at the time we may know little about the injury.

Much depends on the size of the spinal canal. If we have a small canal, or a canal indented into the shape of a pirate's hat, the dura will soon be irritated by the disc, or one of the nerves may even become trapped.

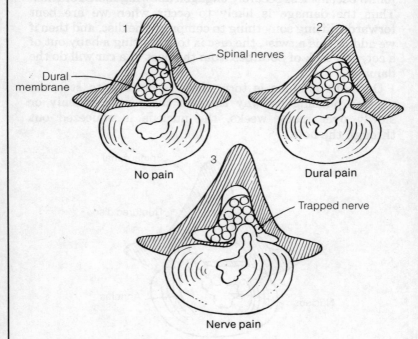

No pain

Dural pain

Nerve pain

What sort of pain is experienced from an injured disc?

If we are going to experience pain from the injured disc, it will first be from the dural irritation, that is irritation of the sheath containing the spinal nerves in their fluid. It produces back pain, and sometimes pain to one side of the back rather than the mid-line. It can even give pain in the buttock or the back of the thigh, and occasionally in the lower abdomen. It can be so severe that we can do no other than lie on the floor, and it may last for hours or weeks.

The dural irritation causes the muscles to go into spasm if we try to bend too far. We may be surprised to find one hip protruding — a result of the same muscle spasm. At times the legs may suddenly give way. They can be alarming symptoms, but are only a protective reaction of the dura rubbing on the protruding disc.

The speed with which these symptoms develop can be very variable. Although for one person the symptoms may be sudden and dramatic, especially if associated with a known injury like slipping, or twisting whilst holding a heavy weight; for another the early stages may be relatively mild, with no more than mild discomfort in the back, or a little ache that is dismissed as a muscle strain. The severity of the symptoms in the early stages depends on the size and the speed of the disc rupture, and the available space in the spinal canal for the nerves to escape harm's way. Some discs bulge very slowly, with a very slow increase in size from minor episodes of stress over several months or even years. It is possible for minor symptoms to come and go, gradually becoming more troublesome until the nucleus of the disc finally ruptures through the outer annulus. Thus these symptoms in the back and perhaps in the buttock from a damaged disc may develop slowly and intermittently for one person, or very suddenly for another.

However, provided a nerve is not trapped we may suffer no more than this type of back pain, with perhaps some muscle spasm making the back stiff or twisted. Whether it developed quickly or slowly, the disc material gradually shrinks; we make a good recovery, perhaps never to be troubled again.

Will other parts of the body be affected by an injured disc?

The disc may not only irritate the dura, but trap a nerve. Symptoms usually start with dural pain — pain in the back; but involvement of a nerve gives pain down the leg below the knee. It generally starts in the buttock, then affects the back of the thigh, or the outer side, then the calf, around the ankle, and at times pins and needles quite distinctly in the big toe or outer foot. It can amount to an ache or a very severe pain. The pain is usually worse when we are standing and walking, and it is relieved by lying down, though not necessarily at once. Again this nerve pain, like the dural pain, can last a short or a long time.

An interesting sign is the inability to sit in the bath with the legs stretched out. The doctor looks for the same sign when the extended leg cannot be lifted very far without pain. He will ask you to lie down, and finds that he cannot lift your heel very far from the bed if the knee is kept straight. It indicates that the nerve is stretched over the protruding disc, and if we try to stretch the nerves further by lifting the leg, it hurts. The nerve runs down the leg behind the knee, and if we relax the nerve by bending the knee, we can lift the leg or sit in the bath comfortably. It is a very clear sign of a trapped nerve.

We know that our likelihood of getting leg pain from a damaged disc depends greatly upon the shape of the spinal canal — the 'important space' discussed on page 12. If we are fortunate enough to have a canal with lots of room, the nerves to the legs are not easily trapped, but a disc bulging into a shallow canal quickly involves one of the nerves, and hence, leg pain.

Will the damaged disc get better and will the pain ever go away?

A disc has been damaged, and we know about it. There is

back-ache, and perhaps pain right down the leg. What will the end of it be? Will there be problems? — Yes and No.

Let's deal with the 'No' first. (We'll deal with the 'Yes' — the problems — in another chapter.)

It is not worth being too pessimistic, because the first attack of disc symptoms usually settle down with time. The chances of getting better by just waiting are great. More than half are better in a week.

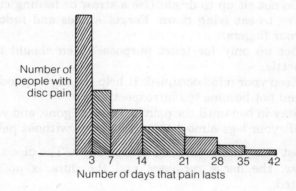

Number of people with disc pain

Number of days that pain lasts

3 7 14 21 28 35 42

Can I influence the outcome?

Discs can probably be made worse by our attempts to cure them. Nature has its own way of trying to put things right, but we are so impatient we can fail to give it a chance. No one has yet shown that there is any better way of relieving disc symptoms than by resting and letting nature take its own course. Pain is a warning sign and should be heeded. Do not struggle on ignoring it. If you do, you will pay double at the end of the day. Lie down and rest, and let your doctor know.

Ten simple rules

1. Go to bed, or put a mattress on the floor and lie on it.
2. Ask someone else to put a strong board under your

mattress — wood not hardboard. A door off its hinges would do.

3. Find a comfortable position, either on your side, or on your back.
4. One pillow should do, and perhaps a pillow under the knees if it eases the pain.
5. Have enough pain relieving tablets to make the pain manageable.
6. Do not sit up to drink. Use a straw or feeding cup.
7. Try to eat lying down. Forget knives and forks. Use your fingers.
8. Get up only for toilet purposes. Men should have a bottle.
9. Keep your mind occupied. It helps to have a good laugh and not become too introspective.
10. Stay in bed until the pain has almost gone, and you can lift your legs almost to a right angle without pain.

Almost everyone eventually settles down. The disc shrinks in size, the nerve recovers, and the dura is no longer irritated.

Can tablets help?

We mentioned this above in one of the 'ten simple rules', suggesting we should have enough pain relieving tablets to make the pain manageable.

If the pain is really so severe we can do no other than lie on the floor in agony, the doctor usually provides strong pain-killing tablets or even an injection. Such tablets should be repeated regularly for the next couple of days, gradually reducing the dose and frequency. We can become too dependent on them, and may suffer from some side effects, but in the early stages of an acute attack, they can give welcome relief. It is not possible to generalise on a programme of tablet-taking, because we are all so different, but it is probably safe advice to take pain relieving tablets to ensure a good night's sleep, and when the acute episode has settled, take tablets in the day only if the pain is not eased by other methods (changing one's position, a pillow under the knees, warmth, a hot bath).

Once we are back on our feet, and still suffer some pain during the day, it is probably more important not to mask the pain symptoms by taking tablets in the day-time. We should be asking why are we getting the pain, and modifying life accordingly. Pain is the body's warning sign of some abuse, and should not be ignored by the ostrich attitude of burying one's head in the sand.

If the pain is not of mechanical origin, but rather associated with an inflammatory disorder (page 52), then a course of anti-inflammatory tablets is useful, but these have little place in the treatment of disc problems.

What happens if in two weeks I am no better?

If pain from a damaged disc has really not settled down in spite of two weeks' strict bed rest at home, it is probably better to go into hospital rather than struggle on at home. Hospital treatment may consist only of further supervised bed rest with adequate sedation, providing a degree of enforced rest that was not proving possible at home. Alternatively, continuous traction may be used in association with bed rest.

What is the effect of traction?

This is not the torture it sounds. It does no more than ensure that the trunk is kept fairly still, to give the lower spine the rest that it needs, whilst still allowing movement of the legs and upper limbs. A corset is applied round the pelvis, with a tape extending on either side down to the foot of the bed fastened to a pulley system over the end of the bed with about 20 lb weight attached. The foot of the bed is slightly raised, so that the body acts as a counter traction. The weights are applied gradually and the patient soon finds it is comfortable, relieving some of the pain. A few patients find that the stomach muscles ache, but a pillow under the knees soon relaxes the stomach. Two weeks of this treatment is often the answer to those who have not settled down at home.

Will I need an operation?

Very occasionally when there is no improvement over several weeks, it is worth having an operation to remove the ruptured piece of disc from the spinal canal. It is usually preceded by a special type of X-ray called a myelogram, when a fluid is injected inside the dura, making it easily seen on X-ray. The ruptured piece of disc is seen indenting the dura. This helps the surgeon to be quite clear which disc is at fault, and makes the operation much simpler, restricting it to the one small area involved. It is a very straightforward operation, removing only the ruptured piece, and clearing other pieces from the centre of the disc. Recovery is usually quite dramatic. Rather than operate, some surgeons are injecting an enzyme into the disc to make it shrink in size, with good results.

What replaces the disc after surgery?

This worries many patients. They feel sure something must be inserted to replace the disc that has been removed. But no — at operation the piece of disc that is protruding through the torn annulus into the spinal canal is gently removed. It is usually found pressing on a nerve, and will often come away very easily in one piece. The hole in the annulus is then explored, and any other pieces of nucleus that could later give trouble if squeezed through the tear are removed. A space is left in the middle of the disc, but this fills with scar tissue. The disc and the adjacent vertebrae slowly change their anatomy in just the same way as an unoperated disc, except that the ruptured piece that was pressing on the nerve has been removed. We have not yet reached the age of plastic discs.

Will it recur?

So this attack has settled down. Will it recur?

You can never be quite sure, because there is always the chance of more attacks. The damaged disc will never be quite the same again, but discs that have been damaged may be symptomless. However, having once injured your back, you should know about the possibilities, and what you can do about it.

Almost anything can happen over the years, but quite a lot of people keep having recurrences of pain from time to time. No one can accurately predict the future, but there are several possibilities.

Can I prevent a recurrence?

You can try. You may not succeed even with the best will in the world, because once damaged, that disc will never be quite the same again. It was there for a purpose, and cannot now function normally. The disc was part of that three joint system (the disc and the two small facet joints at the back) between the two vertebrae. It used to stand up to a lot of strain, but now small mechanical stresses are likely to upset it. However, you should certainly try to prevent a recurrence, even if you are not entirely successful.

Prevention depends upon an understanding of the mechanics of the spine. Let us start with a lever. Only a small force applied a long way from the fulcrum can move a ton. Similarly enormous forces are generated in the lower back when we stoop forwards to pick up a small weight. A normal healthy disc can often cope with these forces — the intact annulus just bulging with the strain — but with a damaged annulus, the pressures generated by a small lift in the stooped position will squeeze out some more of the nucleus through the tear. Even if the damaged disc eventually shrivels up, the anatomy of that area of the spine is now not quite normal, and excessive force can produce problems.

How should I lift?

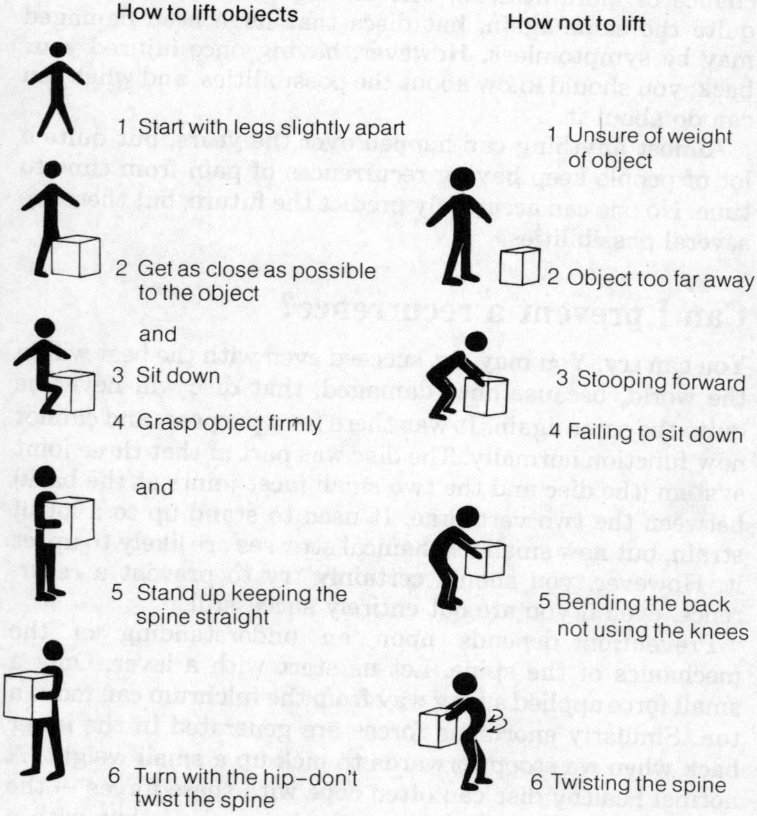

How to lift objects

1 Start with legs slightly apart

2 Get as close as possible to the object

and

3 Sit down

4 Grasp object firmly

and

5 Stand up keeping the spine straight

6 Turn with the hip–don't twist the spine

How not to lift

1 Unsure of weight of object

2 Object too far away

3 Stooping forward

4 Failing to sit down

5 Bending the back not using the knees

6 Twisting the spine

28

Remember the weight lifter and do the same.
Keep your back straight, and in the vertical position,
Keep the weight as close to the body as possible.
Have your feet slightly apart for stability.
Squat down, bend your knees, and do the work with your legs.

Twisting probably caused the first tear of the annulus, and twisting could now finish the job off. It could make a small disc protrusion into a big one. So do not twist your back when it is loaded. When lifting an object from one place to another anticipate the unexpected twist, and have one foot already pointing in the direction you hope to go. You will not then be caught off balance. Move round with your legs rather than with your back. If the weight has to be moved as well as lifted, get some momentum into the activity by using your leg muscles, and be sure your back is kept straight.

Set a limit to the weight you are prepared to lift, and always stick to it. The damage is often done in an unguarded moment when we take a risk. We may think it will save time, but regret it when we are laid up in bed as a result of it. Women alone at home may feel that they have to lift because there is no-one to help. A man may lift because he is embarrassed to be thought weak. However, we often have an instinct about what we can and cannot lift — take note of your senses. Ask for help if it looks too heavy. Get a feel of the weight of an object before you lift it. Gently test it. If it is too heavy, leave it alone. Use a trolley, a barrow, a hoist. Make use of levers. Roll an awkward box along the floor rather than lift it. Divide the load into smaller parts. Take longer over the job. The frequency of lifting a weight is just as important as the weight itself. Move a few boxes. Have a rest and then move some more. Do not try to do it all at once. Invest in a shopping basket on wheels. It all takes a little more time, but it is well worth it.

Be sure that you are wearing the right clothes for the job. It is very difficult for a woman to lift correctly wearing a skirt. Wear trousers if there is lifting to be done. Do not try to lift and carry in your best clothes or you will be automatically trying to keep them clean by holding the object too far from your body instead of clutching it to you. Men should wear overalls when a lifting job is required. See that your pockets are empty or you may suffer a double injury.

How can I remember to lift properly?

Lifting correctly is a motor skill, not easily learnt. Reading this book will not ensure that you lift correctly, any more than reading how to play golf will make a golfer of you. A musician does not learn his technique without recurrent practice, and correction; and neither will you master the ability of correct lifting without much repetitive practice and supervised correction. It helps to have someone else at hand to criticise those everyday activities that might be putting too much stress on your back. Old methods have to be unlearnt, and it will not come easily. This is the area where a good physiotherapist can help you most.

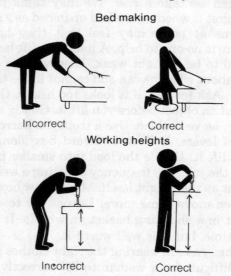

Bed making

Incorrect   Correct

Working heights

Incorrect   Correct

30

Furniture height

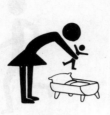

Incorrect   Correct

Working heights

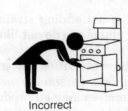   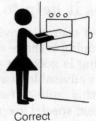

Incorrect   Correct

Pushing

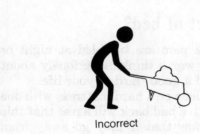   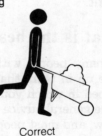

Incorrect   Correct

Walking

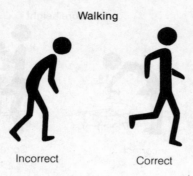

Incorrect   Correct

Does it help to keep fit?

Yes, of course, provided it is not adding strain to the disc. Swimming is the best way, and if you do not like water, then walking is good for you.

It is advisable to avoid those activities that give you pain, and this will differ from one person to another. Golf, jogging, special keep-fit exercises may all produce pain — if that is the case they should be avoided, but if not and you enjoy these activities, carry on with them. They will keep you fit.

What is the best sort of bed?

So many people with back pain are troubled at night or wake up in pain, that it is worth thinking seriously about the bed in which you spend a good third of your life.

The general advice is to sleep on a hard mattress with one pillow, and most people with a bad back will agree that this helps. Conversely, they know that if they go away from home and sleep on a soft sagging mattress, they suffer as a result. No two backs are alike, however, and what is good advice for one is not necessarily right for another. One man I know finds his back is most comfortable if he sleeps in a hammock.

What is best for you is the bed that you can sleep in with

least discomfort, and the majority of us find that this is one with a firm mattress. So many manufacturers are advertising their special orthopaedic mattress that the customer is confused, and as it is such an expensive business you should request a few nights' trial with a mattress before you purchase it.

There are several new designs promising to give relief to the poor back pain sufferer. One is sprung interiorly at pressures that vary from one part of the bed to another, being softer at the level of the shoulders and hips. When you then lie on your side the spine should be straight. Another design relies on laths under the mattress which spring up under the light pressure of the waist and legs, but spring down under the heavier pressure of the shoulders and hips. These designs are excellent in theory, but you will only know if your money is well spent by trying them.

How should I sit?

It can be argued that the sitting posture is vital to a healthy back. It has not been proved that slouching in a chair damaged anyone's back, but those who suffer from back pain know that some chairs are definitely more comfortable than others and that if they neglect their posture their backs will ache. So perhaps if the disc is already damaged posture and chairs are important, but it has yet to be shown that the undamaged back suffers from neglect in the sitting position.

As with the mattress, it is a question of trial and error, but you will probably find that your back is most comfortable in a chair which supports the small of the back, which allows you to take weight evenly along the thighs, and is of a height that allows you to have your feet flat on the floor with ease. You will probably suffer most from a chair that is too low and too soft.

If you work at a desk, its level will also have to be adjusted so that you are not stooping forwards.

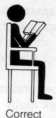

Sitting

Incorrect   Correct

What about car seats?

Travelling long distances in a car will undoubtedly upset
your back. It is probably a combination of vibration, bad
seating, and the inability to control the spine as you veer
from side to side and backwards and forwards on the
journey.

Driving position

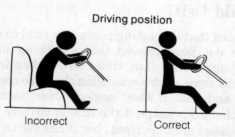

Incorrect   Correct

If you have a choice therefore, you should restrict travel
by road to a sensible minimum. An essential long journey
should be broken up into sections with periods between that
give you the chance to walk about and change your position.

If the choice is not yours, and your job depends on
driving, you must see that the seat is the best you can buy.
Test drive a few cars before purchase. An excellent car seat
has been manufactured that can be adjusted to fit snugly
into any back. You buy the complete seat, fix it into your
new car, and when you change your car, take it with you for
the new vehicle. There are cheaper versions of seat supports

for cars. In an emergency, a rolled up towel in the small of your back can serve very well.

Is standing bad for me?

If you have back pain, you will have learnt that you are better on the move than just standing still. So if your job involves standing for long, find some way out of it. Keep moving about even from one foot to the other, and learn to change the position of your spine when you do stand still, tilting the pelvis forwards and backwards, changing the curve and hollow at the bottom of your back.

If you are in company, do not stand on ceremony, sit down even if others are on their feet. No-one else will look after your back if you do not. Alternatively, it helps to lean against a wall, or sit on the edge of a table. If you are working at the sink or at a bench, purchase a high stool so that you are not standing too long at any one time.

Can anyone help me?

You may say that so far all the advice has been 'self-help'. Rest, wait, be careful and nature will do the rest. Is there no place for positive treatment to speed up the process? If we are talking about the damaged disc in the early days, or even in the subsequent months, you can do no better than leave it alone and let it get better without interference. Attempts to interfere because of impatience may, in fact, make the problem worse.

What about a manipulation?

Well, no-one quite knows what happens when a damaged disc is manipulated. Some say they have 'put your disc back'. It is just conceivable that the disc is sucked back, or that the manipulation tightens up the remaining outer fibres of the annulus and squeezes the partially ruptured disc nucleus back into place. The weakness of the annulus, however, is still there, and with the next strain it could bulge through again. Alternatively, the manipulator may have eased the dura or the nerve away from the protruding disc, and all is well until the nerve or dura find their way back to the same place again. Certainly some patients are helped by a manipulation, but many manipulators would say the manipulation of a damaged disc is risky and would themselves not recommend it. In the process, a small tear of the annulus could be converted into a large tear, and the whole of the central nucleus could rupture through into the spinal canal, with major problems.

Can physiotherapy help?

If you mean exercises, massage, ultrasonics, then the answer is 'no'. Perhaps in the later stages, when we are on the road to recovery, there is a place for physiotherapy to provide muscle-strengthening exercises, but most physiotherapists would keep their hands off a new disc lesion.

This is certainly not to say that the physiotherapist or the manipulator should not be treating back pain. Their practices thrive on recommendations of many who have found considerable help, and both within and outside the Health Service there are expert practitioners who are helping back pain sufferers. However, when dealing with the new disc injury, there are strong grounds for thinking that a manipulation can add further damage to the disc, though perhaps temporarily it gives some relief to symptoms.

Years later, when the old disc injury has produced wear and tear changes, the back is stiff and the joints set, manipulations may be helpful, and certainly for problems further up the spine this treatment can be invaluable. In the early stages, however, try to let the back settle without adding more strain to it, and help yourself.

What about diet?

It may seem at first sight that it would be sensible to lose weight, because all the weight of the upper part of the body is carried on the lower part of the spine. Surely every extra kilogram we carry will be an added force to injure the spine.

If we have increased in weight fairly quickly in past months, this is likely to be in the form of fat, and it is certainly placing added strain on the lower spine. To remove it again makes good sense. If on the other hand we have always been overweight, the spine may have adapted to this, and losing weight may not necessarily be an advantage. Think of the champion weight lifters, and their massive frames, mostly muscle, some fat — to reduce weight for them would be to reduce function.

You could argue that a good healthy layer of muscle and fat around the abdomen produces a firm splint for the lumbar spine, stabilising it when we come to lift.

There is, in fact, no evidence that patients with back-ache are any heavier than the general population.

That is not to say that those who have recently increased their weight, and now experience back pain, should not diet to return to their normal weight. If we have been lying around, getting generally unfit, waiting for back pain to settle down and have steadily increased our girth, this will be an unaccustomed extra burden for the spine to carry, especially when its supportive muscles are not up to tone. This person should diet. Return to the weight you were before the back pain started, and keep it there.

How do you do it? Simply have smaller meals, buy some bathroom scales, and keep a weekly record of progress. If it proves difficult your doctor can provide special dietary advice.

There is a special group of patients with back pain (see pp. 42 and 48) who should take their weight seriously — patients with an unstable spine where some unnatural movement is taking place. But generally weight reduction is only important for the patient with a damaged disc if there has been a sudden recent increase.

How can I take advantage of the situation?

It is rather salutary to be suddenly halted in the middle of a busy life, and we naturally look around for short cuts to a cure. We would be well advised to accept the situation, albeit with our eyes wide open, that healing takes time and requires patience. This is described by Paul the Apostle as a fruit of the Spirit. In the process of waiting we have time to reflect, assess what we are making of life, make a spiritual pilgrimage, and who knows, we may be better persons at the end of the day. The spine has been beautifully designed. Perhaps the Designer has something to say to us if we have time to listen. The pace of life is busy enough. What about making the most of the opportunity to rest, be quiet, relax? Have we recently stepped back to look at the priorities in life? What are we making of it? Should we think about changing course? There can be a bonus in this enforced rest if we look for it. If we are unduly frustrated by our lack of patience, it may be a sign that our lives are too busy, and we have not only been putting too much stress on our backs, but on ourselves.

4. WHAT ARE THE LONG TERM EFFECTS OF DISC INJURY

What happens to the disc over the years?

As the months pass, the damaged disc shrinks in size, and over the years it reduces further, until the two vertebrae which were widely separated by the healthy disc settle much closer together. This takes years to develop and is often without symptoms. We may have forgotten about the old disc pain so many years ago. Did it really put us to bed? The years slip by, and silently the shrivelled disc alters slightly the anatomy of that part of the spine. We are generally quite oblivious of it.

What is arthritis?

We often do not know it is there unless we have an X-ray. As the two vertebrae settle closer together, the small facet joints at the back of the vertebrae alter their position slightly. The upper part of the facet joint sinks into the lower part, and inevitably some 'wear and tear' changes slowly develop in these facet joints. Again this often occurs without any symptoms at all. In a similar way most of us develop some 'wear and tear' changes in the knees or hands as we get older, without any associated pain. These rough patches that develop in our joints may be called 'arthritis' but it is a 'wear and tear' arthritis and nothing at all to do with rheumatism. It is not something that will spread to any other joint, and it is not crippling.

In addition, extra bone develops at the edges of the vertebral bodies. It forms at the front and sides, and occasionally at the back, where the ligaments are attached. It is presumed that the ligaments have to take extra strain following a damaged disc, and this extra bone is evidence of this. Again it may be termed a 'wear and tear' arthritis. It is not at all serious, and we are usually ignorant of its presence.

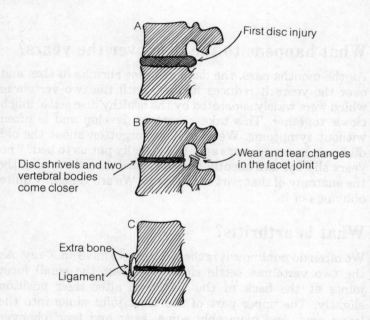

A — First disc injury

Disc shrivels and two vertebral bodies come closer — Wear and tear changes in the facet joint

Extra bone
Ligament

What happens to the old disc rupture?

We may ask, if a nucleus ruptures through a torn annulus into the spinal canal, does it remain in the spinal canal for a lifetime? It probably remains as a thickened piece of scar tissue encroaching a little into the spinal canal, but reduced in size from the time of the original rupture. The nucleus can come through an annular tear like a collar-stud, and it will not go back. But it shrinks and eventually forms scar tissue. If it was previously a symptomless disc injury, it may remain so. If it gave symptoms, it may not give them again. However, for some of us, this scarred disc material can give rise to new symptoms in later life.

How useful are X-rays?

If X-rays show arthritis, or 'wear and tear' changes, that generally does not matter. What, therefore, is the value of an X-ray? Again, X-rays show only the bones, but discs, ligaments and nerves are not visualised at all. So why have X-rays?

The X-rays are only of value to the doctor in trying to put the whole picture together, being interpreted along with all the present and past symptoms, and the examination he makes. Alone, the X-rays do not provide a quick and easy diagnosis.

If a patient is under thirty years of age and has a badly damaged disc, the X-rays are usually quite normal. If he has been born with some slight abnormality in the shape of the spine (and this is commonly present in 5 to 10 per cent of the population) it will show on X-ray, but only be of interest and probably no help.

Once over the age of thirty the X-rays may be useful, because they can show evidence of some injury that occurred a decade before. For instance, we can damage a disc in our early twenties, but the injury may be mild and the canal sufficiently wide for us to escape major problems. Extra bone can begin to form at the edges of the vertebrae on either side of the disc, however, and the two bones may settle closer together. Now in our thirties, a further injury to the disc can cause it to rupture completely with all the symptoms of back and leg pain, and the X-ray will then give a clue to the disc involved.

41

The presence of 'wear and tear' changes on an X-ray can also be helpful when we have pain in the leg and back later in life, but this becomes obvious on page 43 and we are getting ahead of ourselves. Sufficient to say that this is a useful investigation but it needs interpreting in the light of all the factors. To casually talk about 'arthritis of the spine' or 'spondylosis', words which mean only wear and tear changes, does not really help us unless we realise that they gradually develop in most of us and may never cause symptoms at all.

What are the long term effects?

As the vertebrae settle closer together, one important part of the vertebral anatomy changes, and may be a cause of symptoms. This is the tunnel through which a pair of nerves leave the spinal canal on either side and pass into the soft tissues. The nerve tunnel is formed partly by the vertebra above, and partly by the lower vertebra, forming two opposing arches. If the two vertebra come closer together, the tunnel gets smaller and the nerve within, because of less room, becomes very vulnerable. It can be a cause of leg pain (or sciatica) in later life.

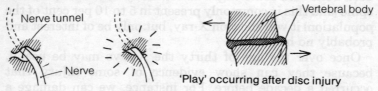

Nerve tunnel

Nerve

Vertebral body

'Play' occurring after disc injury

A second late effect of disc damage is the development of some unnatural movement at that particular level of the spine. The whole spine of vertebrae and discs should move as one unit, like a flexible rod, but after a disc injury some 'play' can occur at that vertebral level. It may only amount to a millimeter or so. For some it is a source of symptoms, for others it matters not at all.

5. WHAT IS SCIATICA?

Sciatica is not pain all over the leg, but pain in a distinct distribution down the leg reaching below the knee. It is pain related to one nerve, and it is felt down the course of that nerve in a clear pattern. It usually affects the buttock, the thigh (back or outer side), the calf, ankle and often the foot (the outer side or the big toe). It can be a pins and needles sensation, an ache or a severe pain. It can start at one place and spread to another.

Years ago it was thought to be due to infection. After the discovery of the disc rupture in 1935, all sciatica was thought to be due to a damaged disc. We now know that sciatica in early adult life is usually due to a disc protruding onto a nerve in the spinal canal, but sciatica in middle life is more often involvement of the nerve at a different site and from a different cause. Certainly disc damage is often responsible, but it is not until perhaps twenty years after disc damage, that the nerve is affected.

How is the nerve damaged?

A disc injury, years before, has altered the anatomy of the nerve tunnel, and the nerve now leaving the spine has less room. Not only has it less room because the two vertebrae have settled closer together, and the tunnel therefore has become smaller, but extra projections of bone from the wear and tear process of the years can protrude into the nerve tunnel and irritate the nerve. In addition, any unnatural movement of the two vertebrae means that the boundaries of the tunnel are moving, and the nerve inside it can be affected. We may be surprised to know that the nerve is rarely stationary; it slides in and out of the tunnel as we move a limb or twist and bend the spine. If the nerve is becoming irritated because of restricted space, it forms a protective covering. A sudden jarring of the back, an awkward twist, some heavy lifting, can be too much for the nerve. Further movement of the nerve in and out of the tunnel irritates it sufficiently to give pain down the length of the nerve. The nerve is being affected at a slightly different site and from a different cause than an early disc injury. The distribution of pain, however, may be the same.

What can I do to alleviate the pain?

The pain can build up to be very severe. It is often constant pain, day and night. It does not seem to be eased by lying down. It is worse sitting or standing for long. Walking far can be difficult. Some patients develop the pain out of the blue, the previous disc trouble having been symptomless because the spinal canal was wide enough. Others remember a disc as a distant memory. Others have had mild manageable back pain. But this new sciatica can be very unpleasant indeed.

Try to discover what positions or activities are painful, and then avoid them. If walking far brings on the pain, do not ignore the warning signs. You will be doing further damage to the nerve. Walk only short distances, within your limits of pain. If it hurts to sit, keep changing your position or lie down. Try to find a comfortable position lying, perhaps with a pillow under your knees, or curled up on your side. Do not travel too far in the car. Protect your back by avoiding heavy lifting and carrying, hoovering, bending and twisting.

If you are in pain in spite of this, an epidural injection can help. This is an injection of salty water into the nerve tunnel, and the pressure of the fluid can free adhesions and loosen up the nerve. Some cortisone in the injection can quieten down an angry nerve, and some local anaesthetic helps.

Some manipulators think they can help this condition, and some physiotherapists believe heavy traction is useful, but these methods have not been scientifically evaluated. An understanding of the cause of the pain, and some practical common sense in trying to manage it, is sufficient for many sufferers to find gradual relief.

Will the sciatica settle down?

If the sciatica has become really troublesome, the chances are that it will not readily go away. One out of four will lose the pain completely within six months, but three out of four will have some discomfort in the leg, on and off, for some years. It does clear eventually.

The lesson to be learned is that sciatic pain in middle life must be taken seriously, and the first warning signs should be heeded. Come off work, rest and do not aggravate it.

6. WHAT IS THE CAUSE OF PERSISTENT BACK PAIN IN MIDDLE LIFE?

We will restrict ourselves to back pain associated with previous disc damage — perhaps many years before — the late effects of which are now producing pain. It is not possible to look into the back and identify the exact source of this pain, but we can make some reasonable suggestions.

Just as the dura can be the source of pain in a new disc protrusion, so also it can cause pain in subsequent years. If the dura is irritated it is well supplied with small nerves especially on its front surface, and this is probably the source of a lot of pain we feel in the back. It may be all across the lower back, or on either side. One side of the back may be more affected than the other; and not only the back — dural irritation can give rise to pain felt in the buttock or even down the back of the thigh. We must consider six factors:

1. A spinal canal which is small in size or indented in shape. This will provide less reserve space for the dura if the spinal canal is compromised in some way. The majority of us have sufficiently wide spinal canals to avoid the problem of persistent back pain even when the back is injured.
2. A previous disc injury. The first symptoms may have cleared, but a disc rupture becomes scarred, taking up

space in the front of the canal. Extra bone may also have formed at the edge of the disc. As the vertebrae settle together, the ligaments can thicken. This leaves a potential problem, of restricted space.

3. A new spinal injury. If the back, which has a small spinal canal and has had a previous disc injury, is now suddenly subjected to a strain, the tight dura can produce pain. An awkward fall can be enough to jar such a back and start off dural pain.

4. The spinal canal has more room when we bend forwards, and less as we lean back. If the dura is already tight, leaning backwards will constrict it further and produce pain. Hence the familiar stooped posture of the back pain sufferer. He will also have difficulty lying face-down in bed, when the arched back is painful.

5. Some vertebrae develop unnatural movement after· a damaged disc with a few millimeters of 'play'. If the dura is already tight, bending and lifting will then give back-ache.

6. It is difficult to be sure how much pain we can get from an arthritic facet joint — that is a joint that has become rough through 'wear and tear'. Certainly these joints develop arthritic changes some years after a disc injury, but very often this can be seen on an X-ray of people with no back pain. No doubt they can give pain that is aggravated by movement.

7. WHAT IS AN UNSTABLE SPINE?

We have mentioned already that the spine should move as a unit. When unnatural movement, or 'play', occurs at one level, this is considered an unstable segment of the spine. It may give pain from upsetting the dura, but the pain could arise in the facet joints from strained ligaments or somewhere else in that segment. Whatever the cause, certain symptoms give it away.

What can cause this?

The back pain is generally worse when we are on our feet, for example, when we are shopping or doing housework; and it improves by lying down for an hour. It gets worse after working in the stooped position for long, such as gardening — when we do come to straighten up again it is difficult. We use our hands to climb up our legs to regain the erect position. In the process we may feel a catch, giving a stab of back pain. You could almost imagine one vertebra, having strained forward a little on the one below, regaining its normal position.

These symptoms are not uncommon in women who first started with back pain in pregnancy. Perhaps the weight of the baby, and the hormones which loosen the ligaments in pregnancy contribute to developing an unstable segment.

Although this instability is not always the result of a disc rupture, it is one of its causes.

X-rays may show evidence of a previous disc injury years ago. It may also show one vertebra displaced forwards or backwards on another. The difficulty for the doctor is that even though this displacement may be quite marked, it can have been present from abnormal growth changes in early life and be quite a stable displaced segment. We will try to make this clearer on page 54.

Can I cure it?

Most people are prepared to live with the pain, and modify their life accordingly to keep it manageable. A corset can help. If you are overweight this certainly needs correction by diet, because every extra kilogram will aggravate the stress on the unstable segment.

Manipulations will increase the problem. In fact, many unstable spines are the late result of repeated manipulations.

Some people favour injections of sclerosing solutions into the tissues at the back of the spine to tighten up the ligaments.

Rarely, an operation to fuse the two unstable vertebrae into one solid piece is worthwhile. It is quite a big operation, but if the diagnosis is correct, and the fusion sound, the results are excellent.

The best advice, unless the pain is very severe, is to come to terms with the pain, altering your life to minimise spinal stress.

Most people know that stooping and lifting in the stooped position aggravates the pain, but a correct lift with a straight back does not. They know that standing too long makes it ache, but leaning on a wall or sitting on a high stool relieves it. They learn to modify shopping expeditions, and are relieved to put their feet up for an hour in the afternoon. Coming to terms with it is not easy, but it may be the only way.

8. DOES PREGNANCY AGGRAVATE BACK PAIN?

No one can accurately predict the effect of pregnancy on back pain. It could make it worse, or it could give relief of the pain. For that reason it is probably sensible for a woman to have a baby irrespective of previous back pain symptoms, but take extra care of the spine for the nine months or more.

We know that generally a woman in pregnancy is twice as likely to develop back pain as a woman the same age not carrying a baby. This is mainly because a hormone is produced by the pregnant mother to soften the ligaments and allow easy passage of the baby through the pelvis. The spinal ligaments are also softened, and with the added weight of the baby in front of the spine, some strain can develop at one vertebral segment, and the spine become 'unstable' at that level.

It is probably aggravated by an excessive hollow developing in the small of the back, the tummy being pushed forwards and the bottom backwards. A shearing force is produced at the very last joint of the spine, with one vertebra straining forwards on another. It is aggravated by wearing high heel shoes. A conscious effort should be made to pull the tummy in and flatten the hollow in the lower back. A special pregnancy corset with an expandable elastic segment in front can also add some support to the spine.

Of course, all the techniques of correct lifting must be

irritation of the eyes. It is more common in young men than women, and research has recently shown that there is a genetic tendency for some of us to be more prone to this disease than others.

It can be relatively mild, affecting the lower part of the back only, or smoulder on and off for years affecting the middle of the back as well, or even the whole spine. As it burns itself out, the back pain usually settles, but the spine is left rather stiff. The inflamed ligaments have been replaced by bone, and the small facet joints become solid.

A stiff spine is not too much of a disability provided it is straight and therefore patients with ankylosing spondylitis are advised to sleep on a hard bed with no pillow so that for at least eight hours a day their backs are not getting used to a bent posture.

Tablets and physiotherapy are a great help, and can keep the condition at bay. The activity of the inflammation can be monitored by a blood test, and these patients are best looked after by a rheumatologist keeping an eye on the progress until it quietens down.

Can blood tests help?

They are useful in excluding other rarer causes of back pain such as ankylosing spondylitis. They will be normal if we are suffering from the commonest cause of back pain resulting from some mechanical strain. If, however, the pain is not related to a mechanical disturbance, but to a more rare inflammatory disease, or to a change in the bones themselves, the blood tests will show this. The pattern of pain with these uncommon disorders of the back are so different from the pain resulting from a mechanical disturbance, that the doctor will generally not need any blood tests to help him. He will be able to make his diagnosis from listening to his patient and from a careful examination.

10. WHAT IS SPONDYLOLISTHESIS?

This sounds a very complicated condition if you have not heard of it before, but it is a genuine state that can cause mechanical back pain. If we have a spondylolisthesis, and we place too much stress on the spine, it can be painful.

It is a displacement of one vertebra forwards on another, usually the very last lumbar vertebra. It used to be called a slipped vertebra, because it was thought that the vertebra had slipped forwards as a result of a strain. It is now known that the displacement occurs very gradually during childhood, and once we stop growing no more displacement occurs. It is not so much a slip, as a growth change. The displacement can be only a couple of millimeters, or so great that one bone slips off the other. And it is common. Six to eight per cent of the population have a spondylolisthesis, usually very mild in degree, and most of them know nothing about it. It is quite painless.

What is the cause of this?

The forces of the spine are resolved in a direction forwards and downwards; but they are restrained by the strong arch of bone at the back of the vertebral bodies, by the facet joints, and by the tough ligaments.

For a spondylolisthesis to take place there must be an

inherent weakness of arch of bone behind the vertebral body. This is supported by the fact that it is more common in certain families and in some races like the Eskimos, and that the weakness can sometimes be clearly seen as a gap in the bone on one side only, without any displacement.

In addition to the inherent weakness there probably needs to be a violent strain to loosen up the weakened tissues. Then slowly, as the child grows, the upper vertebra gradually and silently move into a forward position.

What sort of strain sets it off?

It is usually some violent injury in childhood, often well remembered, such as being thrown from a horse, a fall downstairs, or dropping on the bottom when a chair is pulled away; and is often bad enough to produce bruising and perhaps a few days in bed. Years later, a spondylolisthesis is seen on an X-ray.

Does it matter?

If six to eight per cent of the population have it, and they do not know it is there, presumably for most people it does not matter. We do know, however, that those with this condition are more likely to get a certain type of back pain than the rest of us. They often have an 'instability' type of back pain (p. 48) — that is an intermittent troublesome backache, which is worse walking about, shopping and standing, and eased by lying down.

Pregnancy can upset a spondylolisthesis, and the first symptoms of back pain may start then. Obesity is also a problem if there is an underlying spondylolisthesis.

People with a spondylolisthesis are protected, however, from symptoms of a damaged disc. The disc can be damaged, the one above the spondylolisthesis having to take extra strain, but because the vertebral body slips forward leaving the arch of the spinal canal behind in the process, the spinal canal is actually widened. So even if there is a disc injury and rupture, the nerves in the dural sac have plenty of room to escape out of harm's way. Disc symptoms with these people are very unusual.

As a result of a previous disc injury, the nerve root tunnel can be reduced giving sciatica in middle life. The spondylolisthesis is then only recognised incidently from an X-ray.

The symptoms of 'instability' back-ache and sciatica in middle life are treated in the same way as for other patients (pp 44 and 49), irrespective of the spondylolisthesis. The only difference is that if the pain is really prolonged and very troublesome the results of a spinal fusion, stabilising that part of the spine, are very good indeed.

Could it be prevented?

We have no way at present of spotting young people who are developing a spondylolisthesis. If it is picked up on an X-ray, however, they should be given all possible advice about ways of reducing strain on the spine, in the hope of avoiding trouble in later life. There are certain occupations to be avoided. These people are extremely supple, can put the flat of their hands easily on the floor, and for that reason make good gymnasts. Under the stress of high pressure gymnastics, however, the spine often fails. It would be helpful, therefore, to know if an aspiring gymnast or ballet dancer has a spondylolisthesis before starting on a demanding career, and it would be useful also for the pregnant mother to know if it was present. The same ultrasound scan that shows the baby in the womb can show a spondylolisthesis, and perhaps soon it will be a routine examination for every first pregnancy.

We have no way of knowing how the spondylolisthesis itself can be prevented, but once detected, the symptoms of back pain that may be related to it can be prevented by taking care of the spine.

11. CAN PERSISTENT BACK PAIN AFFECT ONE'S LEGS?

This develops quite commonly in those who have had back pain for many years, but because they find the symptoms rather vague and difficult to describe, they begin to feel that no-one understands them. The discomfort builds up in the legs after walking a certain distance. It affects both legs from the thighs down to the feet. It seems to be all over the legs, aching and numb. They feel tired and heavy, and it is an effort to drag one leg in front of the other. You have to stop and wait a few minutes before the discomfort eases, and then go on again for a while before it starts to build up and force another rest. It helps to lean forwards, lean on a wall, or stoop down pretending to fasten a shoe lace.

The basic problem is that the nerves in the spinal canal have just enough room for comfort at rest, but when you start to walk, they need a little more room, and it is not available. You give them more space when bending forwards, but restrict space when leaning back. For that reason it is easier walking uphill stooping forwards than trying to get down a slope leaning backwards. You could perhaps cycle for miles leaning forwards, but walk no distance at all. The same symptoms can occur in bed, with night cramps, and jumpy legs. One of the problems for the doctor is that there is often little to find when he examines you, but the story will make him suspicious that the spinal canal is tight, and a few investigations will confirm it.

Why are the spinal nerves tight?

1. First of all, you started off life with a narrow canal, perhaps in the bottom ten per cent of the population for canal size. This on its own, of course, would not give trouble unless there was some injury to the spine.
2. Secondly, there has usually been a disc injury or even two discs, which, although they may settle down, leave the canal somewhat reduced in size because of scarred tissue and thickened ligaments.
3. Thirdly, there is then the repeated stress and strain on the back, by lifting and twisting, bending and carrying. There are probably several minor falls and accidents, and in the end the facet joints can become rough and irregular with arthritis, and the affected segment of the spine can become unstable. In combination, these reduce the space available for the dura, and the legs can start to ache.

Can this be investigated?

A conventional X-ray may arouse suspicions of a narrow canal, but it is difficult to be sure. A myelogram X-ray will clinch the diagnosis. The X-ray material in the spinal canal shows up on X-ray, and will show quite clearly if the canal is narrow. There is a way of measuring the canal by ultrasound, which is very simple and painless, quite safe and accurate, but it is not yet available in every hospital. The high frequency sound echoes off the bones, and the time interval between the echoes makes it possible to measure the distance between the reflecting surfaces. It will confirm if a narrow canal is present, and can preclude a myelogram.

Similar symptoms can occur from disease of the arteries. Walking up hills is, then, the problem, and your doctor can soon tell if the pulses in your legs are normal or not.

Can this be treated?

The treatment is an operation to remove some of the bone at the back of the spinal canal, making more room for the nerves in the dural sac of spinal fluid. Probably the spinal fluid is the most important factor, and allowing the nerves to bathe in more fluid gives immediate relief of symptoms. This fluid brings nutrients to the nerves, and carries away waste products. If the dura is so tight that the waste products cannot escape, the nerves will not function correctly until we stop to give the nerves a rest, and lean forwards to make more room for the fluid to trickle through the tight space. An operation relieves this tightness, and the cure is usually dramatic.

The operation is fairly simple, and you are home in two weeks.

Are there any after effects?

The spine is still quite stable after the operation because the three joint system is still intact. Only the bone at the back of the spinal canal has been removed. In fact, some of us are born with this bone missing (a spina bifida occulta), and are not aware of its absence. The spine is not made weaker by the operation, but there can be some difficulties after the operation, due to the formation of scar tissue. It is not uncommon for the first excellent results to be spoilt by a slow recurrence of the same symptoms again. Scar tissue can form over the operation area, gradually tightening up the dura again. It does not always occur, and it may only produce mild symptoms, but it is common enough to make the surgeon hesitate before operating.

Could I live with these symptoms?

About three out of four with these symptoms do live with them. They take life at a more leisurely pace, do not walk so far, and get no worse. They find symptoms can vary from day to day and with the time of day, and with careful restraint, they learn to cope very well. A few anti-inflammatory tablets can help, but should not be continued if there is no obvious benefit. For most it is either an operation or nothing, and the decision about an operation rests on how severely disabled you are. For those in a lot of trouble, there are bright prospects surgically, but it is fair comment that a few do develop the same symptoms again. Most who have had the operation say it was worth it.

Could the pain be imaginary?

For those who have never experienced it, back pain can be a joke. It is all too easy to say it is only an excuse to be off work, or a reason to receive a bit of sympathy; and those who suffer the pain all too quickly feel the taunts that they must be making the most of the pain, and much of it is imaginary. Soon the patient himself begins to question if some of the pain is 'in his mind' and he can become both muddled and depressed.

The whole concept by which we feel pain is still a mystery, but it is a developing science, and worth thinking about in the context of back pain. First of all, the way we behave to an injury can vary from one day to another, depending on outward circumstances. One man can lose a limb in battle and hardly feel the pain, so involved is he in the conflict. The same injury in another situation produces a different response. Similarly when we visit the dentist, the tooth-ache has gone away, but the source of pain remains. So our behaviour can depend very much upon the surrounding circumstances.

The same source of pain in the spine may produce a variable pain response depending on many outside factors. To mention a few — the pressures at home and at work, our motivation to be fit, or the lack of it, the prospect of reward from litigation if the back injury occurred in an accident, the pleasure of receiving sympathy — all can influence our experience of pain. The pain is not imaginary. It is felt as very real pain, but the intensity with which we feel it, and the behaviour it produces in us is influenced by all manner of external effects.

The basic cause of the pain, however, remains, whether we make much or little of it. It is this basic cause that we are trying to understand in this book, and hopefully as we come to understand more about it, our fears and worries can be reduced, and the very intensity of the pain we experience reduced also.

12. PREVENTION

What of my children?

It is unfortunate but true that man often only learns from
his mistakes. You have had back pain, perhaps only the first
signs of a damaged disc; or maybe the years have gone by
and you are suffering from the late effects of that disc
injury. Had you known how to respect your back in the
beginning you would have taken such care. Had you
anticipated the effects of repeated stress and strain on that
damaged disc with all the late problems that follow, you
would have lived differently. If you cannot help yourself,
can your experience help someone else?

What advice is there to be given for those at risk?

We do know that back problems run in families, so pass on
some sensible advice to your offspring. See that they grow
up with a healthy respect for the spine. We know also that
those with narrow spinal canals are at particular risk. How
can these be identified? There is a new technique using
ultrasound which will quickly measure the spinal canal
without any risk or any pain. Unfortunately, it is not
universally available. There is also a method showing

promise called nuclear magnetic resonance, which only uses magnetism and a radio receiver to show a picture of the spine, but this is still in the development stage. We are beginning, however, to find ways of identifying those at risk. Perhaps until we are more confident, we should provide good advice to all young people, and make them more conscious of the risks they run by abusing their spine.

To protect the disc we would reinforce the advice that lifting and twisting is dangerous. For those at risk, or those already with symptoms, heavy manual work and the stressful sporting and recreational activities should be avoided.

The spine is a marvel of design, supporting the body, allowing movement, protecting the complex nervous system, but there is a limit to its strength. This we must recognise and come to terms with, if we are to live in comfort with our back.

Could I have prevented it?

Many of us would like to put back the clock and make a new start. With the disc this is not possible. We naturally ask the question 'Could it have been prevented?' — at least to be able to pass on advice to our children.

Looking again at the cause of disc symptoms, there are at least *three* recognisable factors that ultimately produce pain.

1. An inherent weakness of the disc making some people more prone than others to develop a tear.
2. A twisting force applied to a loaded disc will tear the weak area of the annulus allowing the nucleus to bulge through.
3. A spinal canal small enough or of such a shape that the nerves within the dura have little room to get out of harm's way.

Factors one and three are probably inherited, and we can do little about them. We should have chosen our parents more carefully!

Factor two is up to us. But it is too late. The damage is done. We can, however, seek ways of warning those with a family history of disc trouble that they are particularly at risk, and inform all young people of the limitations of our spine, and that we abuse it at our cost. Only those who have themselves suffered are likely to be sufficiently motivated, and that means you.

Can back pain be prevented at work?

Low back pain is now the major cause of sickness absence in our heavy labouring industries. It is a problem also amongst sedentary workers, but a much smaller problem. It seems obvious that if the factory can be made as safe for the spine as the office, we can make big inroads into the problem of back pain in industry. The employer must ensure that the job is suited to the man. An enormous volume of research effort is at present expended on safe industrial design, but its application is frequently wanting. The employee must press for safety for his own sake. Men and women are still lifting unacceptable loads through their own and their employer's ignorance. All too frequently they will ignore what lifting aids are available. Work design, however, can reduce the problem.

Can back pain be prevented by education?

Education has little value unless it changes behaviour. There is little evidence to show that the occasional lecture on how to look after your back actually influences a man who has never had back pain. He continues to lift, in the same dangerous manner, loads likely to damage a disc. Habits learnt from childhood are not easily changed, and he lifts, twists and carries loads that still place his back at risk. Only if education changes his behaviour is there a chance of the first disc injury being avoided. It requires demonstration, practice, criticism, repetitive practice and group criticism, until pride in correct handling of materials is a strong enough motivation for a man or woman to see that they always lift correctly, and that they instinctively think out the application of principles of lifting to every new situation. Only then is there a chance that education can reduce the problem of back pain before the first injury has occurred. And how young should we begin? Who should ideally educate? Perhaps teachers of physical education have a unique opportunity, and also parents.

Once we have experienced back pain, we are well motivated to apply all we can learn about reducing stress on the spine. Education is well received and will alter behaviour, but although it can reduce the chance of recurrences of pain, the damage has been done, and there is now a potentially weak area of the spine. Ideally we should be seeking to prevent the first injury.

Can back pain be prevented by screening?

Looking to the future, this would seem to hold out the best chance of reducing the problem. Some of us are obviously at greater risk than others from the start. One man can abuse his back throughout his working life and never have back-ache, whilst another who appears to have led a quiet life is troubled with pain. Can we therefore identify the man at risk, even in his teens; spend our major efforts on 'educating' him about his back and ensure that he is placed in an occupational situation relatively safe for his spine?

We know the size and shape of the spinal canal is a risk factor, and it can be measured by a simple safe ultrasound technique. It is premature to advocate universal screening, because our skills in education to affect behaviour are not established, and because so few industries are really sure which areas of employment are at risk. Automation is producing fewer 'light jobs', and screening may therefore mean unemployment for some who have largely manual skills. The effect of screening on the complex psychological aspect of pain is still ill understood, and therefore although screening to place the right man in the job, where heavy work is unavoidable, offers the best hope for the future, its present general application is premature.

If you are one who suffers from back pain, this book may have given you some food for thought, perhaps explained what is happening to your back, and how you can live with it. We began with the analogy of an intrepid explorer struggling through an uncharted undergrowth. I hope you have now found a more comfortable path, with some daylight ahead.

UNDERSTANDING BACK PAIN

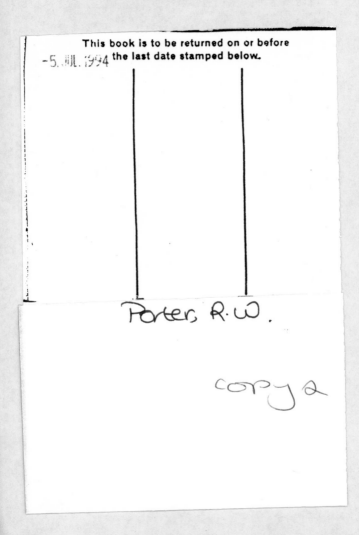